THE UNBREAKABLE LINK BETWEEN EXERCISE AND MENTAL HEALTH

Table of Contents

Chapter 1

Introduction

The thread of mental health runs through every aspect of our lives, influencing the colors and patterns of our experiences. It is crucial to reflect on the significance of mental well-being, especially now. Welcome to "The Unbreakable Link Between Exercise and Mental Health," where we explore the dynamic interplay between the mind and body, and the transformative potential of physical activity.

A. Brief Overview of the Significance of Mental Health

Mental health is the bedrock upon which our emotional, psychological, and social well-being rests. It is the silent conductor orchestrating the symphony of our thoughts, feelings, and behaviors. The significance of mental health extends beyond individual well-being; it is the cornerstone of healthy communities and societies. As we embark on this journey, let us collectively acknowledge and prioritize the intrinsic value of a sound and resilient mind.

B. The Prevalence of Mental Health Issues in Today's Society

In the backdrop of our fast-paced and demanding world, mental health issues have become pervasive, affecting individuals from all walks of life. Anxiety disorders, depression, and stress-related conditions cast shadows across our communities, demanding our attention and collective effort. This ebook seeks to shine a light on the prevalence of these challenges, fostering a compassionate understanding of the struggles many face and the urgent need for effective solutions.

C. Introduction to the Central Theme

1. The Link Between Exercise and Mental Well-being

Amidst the complexities of mental health, a beacon of hope emerges—a link between exercise and mental well-being that has the potential to transform lives. This central theme is the heartbeat of our exploration. In the chapters that follow, we will delve into the depths of mental health, unravel the neurobiological mysteries that connect exercise and the brain, and discover the myriad physical and psychological benefits that await those who choose to embrace a more active lifestyle.

This is an invitation to a journey of self-discovery and empowerment a journey where the rhythmic cadence of your steps mirrors the harmonious dance of a healthier mind. As we venture into the chapters that lie ahead, let us embark on this transformative odyssey together, exploring the intricate and profound connection between exercise and mental health.

Continue to explore the chapters listed below for a comprehensive guide.

Chapter 2

Understanding Mental Health

In the vast landscape of human experience, the contours of our mental health shape the narrative of our lives. Understanding mental health is a pivotal step on our journey to discovering the profound connection between exercise and our psychological well-being.

A. Definition of Mental Health

Mental health is not a static state but a dynamic continuum that encompasses our emotional, psychological, and social well-being. At its core, mental health reflects our ability to cope with the challenges of life, navigate relationships, and make decisions. It is the equilibrium from which resilience, self-esteem, and a sense of purpose emanate.

In this chapter, we will explore a comprehensive definition of mental health that goes beyond the mere absence of mental disorders. Mental health encompasses positive attributes of emotional well-being, such as robust coping mechanisms, emotional intelligence, and the capacity for joy.

As we embark on this exploration, let us reframe our understanding of mental health as a state of flourishing, where individuals can thrive and embrace life's challenges with resilience.

B. Common Mental Health Challenges

As we navigate the complexities of the 21st century, we find ourselves confronting an array of common mental health challenges that transcend age, gender, and cultural boundaries. Understanding these challenges is essential in fostering empathy, reducing stigma, and creating a foundation for meaningful dialogue.

1. Anxiety Disorder

Anxiety, a natural stress response, becomes a disorder when it interferes with daily life. Generalized anxiety disorder, panic disorder, and social anxiety are among the manifestations that impact millions globally.

2. Depression

Depression is more than just fleeting sadness; it is a pervasive sense of hopelessness and despair that affects one's thoughts, feelings, and daily functioning. It is a global burden that requires nuanced understanding.

3. Stress-Related Conditions

In the relentless pace of modern life, stress has become a ubiquitous companion. Chronic stress can lead to various physical and mental health issues, including cardiovascular problems and mood disorders.

4. Importance of Addressing Mental Health Proactively

Proactively managing our mental health is similar to taking preventive care for our minds. By identifying the early signs of mental health challenges and creating a supportive and understanding environment, we can work together to reduce the impact of these issues.

As we move forward, let us develop a compassionate awareness of the various mental health challenges that people face. By understanding the intricacies of mental health, we can lay the foundation for the transformative potential that exercise has in promoting a resilient and flourishing mind.

In the chapters that follow, we will explore the intricate web of connections between exercise and mental health, uncovering how physical activity can serve as a powerful tool for both prevention and intervention in the realm of mental well-being.

Chapter 3

The Science Behind the Connection

In the intricate dance between the body and the mind, the third chapter of our exploration unveils the symphony of the neurobiological impact of exercise on the brain. As we embark on this scientific journey, we uncover the remarkable ways in which physical activity becomes a catalyst for profound changes within the very organ that governs our thoughts, emotions, and well-being.

A. Exploration of the Neurobiological Impact of Exercise on the Brain

1. Understanding Endorphins and Their Role in Mood Regulation

The connection between exercise and mental health is based on the release of endorphins, which are natural mood elevators produced by our body. When we engage in physical activity, these endorphins flood our system, creating a feeling of euphoria and well-being. This natural high not only enhances our mood but also acts as a powerful stress reliever.

2. Effects on Neurotransmitters such as Serotonin and Dopamine

Exercise emerges as a dynamic regulator of neurotransmitters, such as serotonin and dopamine, key players in mood regulation. The surge in serotonin levels contributes to an improved mood and a sense of calm, while elevated dopamine levels enhance feelings of pleasure and reward. This intricate interplay forms the foundation of the mood-enhancing effects of exercise.

3. Impact on Brain Structure and Function

The brain is a highly adaptable organ that can change in response to its environment. Exercise is a powerful stimulant for positive changes in the brain. Physical activity has been linked to increased neuroplasticity, which is the brain's ability to reorganize itself. Regions of the brain that are associated with cognitive function, memory, and emotional regulation show structural improvements, which can lead to improved mental well-being.

By examining the neurobiological mechanisms at play, we can better understand the profound impact of exercise on the brain's chemistry and structure. The complex interplay between endorphins, neurotransmitters, and structural adaptations reveals the science behind the well-known phrase: a healthy body leads to a healthy mind.

In the upcoming chapters, we will continue to unravel the layers of this connection, exploring how exercise becomes a powerful prescription for mental health, offering both preventive and therapeutic benefits. The science behind this connection serves as a testament to the profound synergy between physical activity and our brain's intricate mechanisms. As we deepen our understanding, we equip ourselves with the knowledge needed to embark on a transformative journey toward mental well-being through the simple yet powerful act of exercise.

Chapter 4

Benefits of Exercise for Mental Health

In the ongoing exploration of the profound connection between exercise and mental well-being, this chapter unveils the diverse tapestry of benefits that physical activity weaves for both the body and the mind. From tangible physical enhancements to subtle yet powerful psychological transformations, the benefits of exercise illuminate the path toward a resilient and flourishing mental state.

A. Physical Benefits

1. Stress Reduction

Exercise serves as a natural stress reliever, acting as a counterbalance to the demands of daily life. Physical activity triggers the release of stress hormones, promoting a state of relaxation and easing tension. Regular exercise thus becomes a potent antidote to the pressures that can accumulate in the modern world.

2. Improved Sleep Patterns

Quality sleep is a cornerstone of mental well-being, and exercise plays a pivotal role in fostering restful nights. The calming effects of physical activity, coupled with the regulation of circadian rhythms, contribute to improved sleep patterns. As sleep quality is enhanced, so too does our mental resilience.

3. Increased Energy Levels

Paradoxically, expending energy through exercise leads to increased overall energy levels. Regular physical activity enhances cardiovascular health, oxygenating the body and brain more efficiently. This heightened vitality not only combats feelings of fatigue but also positively impacts our cognitive functions.

B. Psychological Benefits

1. Reduction in Symptoms of Anxiety and Depression

Exercise emerges as a potent ally in the battle against anxiety and depression. The release of endorphins and the modulation of neurotransmitters contribute to a more stable and positive mood. Over time, consistent exercise has been shown to alleviate symptoms associated with these prevalent mental health challenges.

2. Enhanced Cognitive Function

The benefits of exercise extend beyond the physical realm into the cognitive domain. Regular physical activity has been linked to improvements in memory, attention, and overall cognitive function. The brain's ability to process information efficiently is heightened, fostering mental clarity and acuity.

3. Boosted Self-esteem and Confidence

Physical activity cultivates a sense of accomplishment and mastery, which, in turn, enhances self-esteem and confidence. Achieving fitness goals, whether big or small, contributes to a positive self-image and a belief in one's capabilities for a transformative journey from body to mind.

As we navigate the terrain of physical and psychological benefits, we witness the holistic impact of exercise on mental health. The synergy between the body and mind becomes increasingly evident, revealing that the pursuit of a healthier mind is intricately linked to the maintenance of a healthy body. In the chapters ahead, we will explore how different forms of exercise can be tailored to specific mental health goals, offering a roadmap to personalized well-being.

Chapter 5

Tailoring Exercise to Mental Health Needs

As we continue our exploration of the profound interplay between exercise and mental well-being, this chapter unveils the personalized approach to physical activity. Understanding that mental health needs are diverse and nuanced, we delve into the specific types of exercise that align with distinct mental health goals. Moreover, we embark on the journey of creating personalized fitness plans, recognizing that individuality is the key to unlocking the transformative potential of exercise.

A. Types of Exercise for Specific Mental Health Goals

1. Aerobic Exercise for Mood Enhancement

Aerobic activities, such as running, brisk walking, or cycling, stand as powerful mood enhancers. These exercises stimulate the release of endorphins, providing a natural boost to one's mood. Engaging in aerobic exercise regularly has been associated with a reduction in symptoms of anxiety and depression, making it a valuable tool in the pursuit of mental well-being.

2. Strength Training for Stress Relief

Strength training exercises, involving resistance and muscle engagement, offer unique benefits for stress relief. These activities not only build physical strength but also contribute to a sense of empowerment and control. The physical exertion involved in strength training aids in dissipating stress, promoting a calm and centered state of mind.

3. Mind-Body Exercises (Yoga, Meditation) for Relaxation

Mind-body exercises, including yoga and meditation, emphasize the connection between physical movement and mental focus. These practices foster relaxation, alleviate tension, and enhance mindfulness. The incorporation of breathwork in these exercises further contributes to stress reduction and a tranquil mental state.

B. Creating Personalized Fitness Plans Based on Individual Mental Health Needs

1. Assessment of Individual Mental Health Needs

Recognizing that mental health needs vary from person to person, the first step in creating a personalized fitness plan is a thorough assessment of individual requirements. This may involve considering current mental health challenges, personal goals, and preferences in physical activity.

2. Incorporating Enjoyable Activities

A crucial aspect of creating a sustainable fitness plan is the inclusion of activities that individuals genuinely enjoy. Whether it's dancing, hiking, or team sports, finding joy in exercise is essential for long-term adherence. Enjoyable activities not only promote consistency but also contribute to the overall positive experience of physical activity.

3. Setting Realistic and Achievable Goals

Personalized fitness plans should be built on realistic and achievable goals that align with individual mental health needs. Setting milestones that are challenging yet attainable ensures a sense of accomplishment, boosting self-esteem and motivation.

4. Adapting to Changing Mental Health Dynamics

Mental health is dynamic, and individual needs may evolve. A personalized fitness plan should be flexible enough to adapt to changing circumstances, accommodating fluctuations in mood, energy levels, and overall mental well-being.

In the chapters ahead, we will delve deeper into the practical strategies for overcoming common barriers to exercise, ensuring that individuals can implement and sustain their personalized fitness plans. As we tailor exercise to meet individual mental health needs, the transformative potential of this connection becomes a personalized journey toward well-being.

Chapter 6

Overcoming Barriers to Exercise

In the pursuit of a healthier mind through exercise, it's essential to address the common challenges that may hinder the establishment of a regular exercise routine. This chapter focuses on understanding these challenges and provides practical strategies to overcome the barriers, ensuring a sustainable and fulfilling journey toward improved mental well-being.

A. Common Challenges to Maintaining a Regular Exercise Routine

1. Lack of Motivation

Motivation can be elusive, especially when faced with the demands of daily life. Lack of motivation often stems from a disconnect between long-term goals and immediate desires. Recognizing this challenge is the first step toward finding sustainable solutions.

2. Time Constraints

Modern life is often characterized by a hectic pace, leaving little room for additional activities. Finding time for exercise can be a persistent challenge, and individuals may feel overwhelmed by conflicting priorities. Addressing time constraints requires strategic planning and a realistic approach to time management.

3. Physical Limitations

Physical limitations, whether due to existing health conditions or perceived fitness levels, can pose a significant barrier to exercise. Fear of injury or discomfort may deter individuals from engaging in physical activity, necessitating an understanding of personal capabilities and gradual progression.

B. Practical Strategies to Overcome These Barriers

1. Setting Realistic Goals

Establishing realistic and achievable goals is fundamental to overcoming barriers. Break down larger objectives into smaller, manageable milestones. This not only makes progress tangible but also boosts confidence and motivation.

2. Incorporating Physical Activity into Daily Life

Integrate exercise seamlessly into daily routines. This can include simple changes like taking the stairs, walking during breaks, or opting for active commuting. By making physical activity a natural part of daily life, the barrier of time constraints becomes more surmountable.

3. Finding Enjoyable Activities

Engaging in activities that bring joy is a powerful motivator. Experiment with different forms of exercise to discover what resonates personally. When exercise is enjoyable, it transforms from a perceived chore to a rewarding experience.

4. Establishing a Support System

Enlist the support of friends, family, or exercise buddies. A supportive network can provide motivation, encouragement, and accountability. Sharing the journey with others creates a sense of community, making it easier to overcome obstacles.

5. Creating a Consistent Routine

Establishing a consistent exercise routine helps overcome the challenge of motivation. Set specific times for physical activity, creating a structured schedule that aligns with personal preferences. Consistency builds habits, making exercise an integral part of daily life.

6. Adapting to Personal Preferences

Tailor the exercise routine to individual preferences. Whether it's outdoor activities, group classes, or solo workouts, adapting to personal likes and dislikes fosters a sense of ownership and enjoyment.

In the upcoming chapters, we will explore real-life case studies and personal stories to illustrate how individuals have successfully overcome barriers to exercise, highlighting the universal nature of these challenges and the diverse ways in which they can be conquered. As we navigate these strategies, the path to a regular exercise routine becomes clearer, guiding individuals toward a harmonious relationship between physical activity and mental well-being.

Chapter 7

Case Studies and Personal Stories

In the symphony of the mind-body connection, real-life stories resonate as powerful melodies, each echoing the transformative impact of exercise on mental health. This chapter delves into the personal narratives of individuals who have navigated the challenges of mental well-being and found solace, resilience, and renewal through the embrace of physical activity.

A. Real-life Examples of Individuals Who Have Experienced Mental Health Improvements Through Exercise:

1. Sarah's Journey from Anxiety to Empowerment

Sarah, a young professional, grappled with overwhelming anxiety that cast shadows over her daily life. Through the consistent practice of yoga and mindfulness exercises, she not only found relief from anxiety symptoms but also discovered a profound sense of empowerment. Her story underscores the transformative power of mind-body exercises in cultivating mental resilience.

2. James' Battle with Depression and the Marathon of Recovery

James faced the deep abyss of depression, feeling trapped in a cycle of despair. His journey towards mental health involved embracing running, culminating in the remarkable achievement of completing a marathon. The discipline, focus, and sense of accomplishment gained through running became pillars of his recovery, illustrating the ability of aerobic exercise to combat depression.

B. Diverse Stories to Illustrate the Universality of the Connection

1. Maria's Dance

Maria, a mother of three, found solace in dance as a form of self-expression and stress relief. Her story illustrates that the benefits of exercise are not confined to a specific demographic. Regardless of age or background, the joy and liberation found in the movement contribute to enhanced mental well-being.

2. Ahmed's Team Sports and Social Connection

Ahmed, a college student, battled feelings of isolation and anxiety. Joining a team sport not only provided a physical outlet but also fostered a sense of camaraderie and social connection. His story emphasizes the social dimensions of exercise and its role in building a supportive community.

As we immerse ourselves in these stories, it becomes evident that the connection between exercise and mental health is a universal thread that weaves through diverse lives. These narratives serve as beacons of hope, illustrating that the path to mental well-being through physical activity is not exclusive but inclusive—a journey open to individuals from all walks of life.

In the subsequent chapters, we will explore collaborative approaches between mental health professionals and fitness experts, emphasizing the integration of exercise into holistic mental health treatment plans. The stories shared in this chapter lay the groundwork for understanding the multifaceted nature of mental health improvements through exercise, highlighting the potential for transformative change in the lives of many.

Chapter 8

Integrating Exercise into Mental Health Treatment

In the evolution of mental health treatment, harmonious integration of exercise emerges as a dynamic force, reshaping traditional paradigms and offering holistic approaches that extend beyond the therapist's couch. This chapter delves into collaborative models, where mental health professionals and fitness experts work hand in hand, and explores the pivotal role of exercise within comprehensive, holistic mental health treatment plans.

A. Collaborative Approaches Between Mental Health Professionals and Fitness Experts

1. The Therapist-Fitness Expert Alliance

Within this collaborative framework, mental health professionals and fitness experts form a synergistic alliance, recognizing that the mind and body are interconnected. Therapists provide insights into the psychological needs of individuals, while fitness experts contribute expertise in tailoring exercise regimens to align with mental health goals. This multidisciplinary approach offers clients a comprehensive understanding of their well-being.

2. Coordinated Treatment Plans

Collaboration extends beyond mere communication; it involves the creation of coordinated treatment plans. Therapists and fitness experts collaboratively design interventions that seamlessly blend psychological strategies with targeted physical activities. This coordination ensures that individuals receive tailored support addressing both their mental health challenges and their unique physical needs.

B. The Role of Exercise in Holistic Mental Health Treatment Plans:

1. Exercise as a Complementary Therapy

Exercise is positioned as a complementary therapy within holistic mental health treatment plans. It becomes an integral component alongside traditional therapeutic modalities, contributing to a more comprehensive and nuanced approach to mental health care. The combination of talk therapy and targeted exercise creates a holistic environment that addresses the complexity of mental well-being.

2. Targeting Specific Mental Health Goals

Holistic mental health treatment plans leverage exercise to target specific mental health goals. Whether alleviating symptoms of anxiety, enhancing mood stability, or promoting stress resilience, the tailored integration of exercise addresses the diverse needs of individuals. This targeted approach acknowledges the individuality of mental health challenges and aligns interventions accordingly.

3. Long-Term Well-being and Prevention

Beyond immediate symptom relief, holistic mental health treatment plans focus on long-term well-being and prevention. Regular physical activity is positioned as a sustainable, ongoing strategy for maintaining mental health. The emphasis shifts from crisis intervention to proactive measures, fostering resilient and enduring mental well-being.

As we navigate the landscape of integrated mental health treatment, it becomes evident that exercise is not merely an adjunct but a cornerstone of comprehensive care. The collaboration between mental health professionals and fitness experts paves the way for innovative, person-centered interventions that recognize and address the interconnected nature of mind and body. In the chapters to come, we will explore practical tips for readers, guiding them in getting started with an exercise routine and incorporating physical activity into their daily lives. This transition from theory to practical application empowers individuals to take charge of their mental health journey, recognizing exercise as a powerful tool in the pursuit of well-being.

Chapter 9

Practical Tips for Readers

In the pursuit of a healthier mind through exercise, practical guidance becomes the compass that navigates the journey from intention to action. This chapter is a roadmap, offering readers tangible tips to not only initiate their exercise routine but also ensure that it becomes a sustainable and enjoyable part of their daily lives.

A. Getting Started with an Exercise Routine

1. Start Small and Gradual

The journey begins with small, manageable steps. Start with activities that align with your current fitness level and gradually increase intensity. This approach minimizes the risk of burnout and enhances long-term adherence.

2. Choose Activities You Enjoy

Explore various forms of exercise to discover what resonates with you. Whether it's dancing, hiking, or a team sport, engaging in activities you genuinely enjoy makes the initiation phase more enjoyable and sustainable.

B. Setting Realistic Goals

1. Define Clear and Achievable Objectives

Set clear and achievable goals that align with your mental health aspirations. Whether it's improving mood, reducing stress, or building resilience, having specific objectives provides direction and motivation.

2. Break Goals into Smaller Milestones

Break larger goals into smaller, manageable milestones. This not only makes progress tangible but also celebrates achievements along the way. Recognizing small victories contributes to a positive mindset and reinforces the habit of regular exercise.

C. Incorporating Physical Activity into Daily Life

1. Integrate Exercise into Daily Routines

Identify opportunities to incorporate exercise seamlessly into your daily life. This can include opting for stairs instead of elevators, walking during breaks, or scheduling short workouts during pockets of available time.

2. Create a Consistent Schedule

Establishing a consistent exercise schedule enhances the likelihood of adherence. Whether it's morning walks, lunchtime yoga, or evening workouts, consistency fosters the development of habits, making exercise a natural part of your routine.

D. Making Exercise Enjoyable and Sustainable

1. Explore Varied Activities

Keep exercise engaging by exploring a variety of activities. This not only prevents monotony but also ensures that you discover forms of physical activity that resonate with your preferences.

2. Involve Social Elements

Exercise can be a social activity. Involve friends, and family, or join group classes to create a supportive community. The social aspect adds an enjoyable dimension to exercise, making it more likely to be sustained over time.

3. Set Realistic Expectations

Embrace the journey with realistic expectations. Understand that progress may be gradual, and setbacks are a natural part of the process. Setting realistic expectations fosters a positive and sustainable approach to exercise.

As readers embark on their journey of integrating exercise into their lives, these practical tips serve as a compass, guiding them through the initial phases and ensuring that exercise becomes a transformative and enduring companion on their path to mental well-being. The chapters that follow will delve into the conclusion, emphasizing key takeaways and encouraging readers to embrace the empowering potential of exercise in fostering a healthier mind.

Conclusion

Empowering Your Mental Health Journey

As we reach the culmination of our exploration into the profound connection between exercise and mental well-being, let us reflect on the key insights that have illuminated the pages of this journey and consider the empowering potential that exercise holds for the mind.

A. Recap of the Key Points

1. Mind-Body Synergy

We began by recognizing the intricate synergy between the mind and body, understanding that their connection forms the foundation of holistic well-being.

2. Scientific Underpinnings

Delving into the science behind the connection, we explored the neurobiological impact of exercise on the brain, unraveling the release of endorphins, the modulation of neurotransmitters, and the structural enhancements that contribute to mental resilience.

3. Diverse Benefits

From physical enhancements like stress reduction, improved sleep, and increased energy levels to psychological transformations such as reduced anxiety and depression symptoms, enhanced cognitive function, and boosted self-esteem—exercise emerged as a catalyst for holistic well-being.

4. Tailoring Exercise

We navigated the landscape of tailoring exercise to specific mental health needs, understanding the nuanced benefits of aerobic exercise, strength training, and mind-body exercises. Personalized fitness plans were revealed as the compass guiding individuals toward their unique well-being goals.

5. Overcoming Barriers

Recognizing common challenges and providing practical strategies, we dismantled the barriers that often hinder the establishment of a regular exercise routine, paving the way for sustained engagement in physical activity.

6. Real-life Narratives

Through case studies and personal stories, we witnessed the universal nature of the connection between exercise and mental health. These narratives underscored that regardless of background or circumstance, individuals have found solace, strength, and renewal through the transformative power of physical activity.

7. Integration into Treatment Plans

The collaborative integration of exercise into mental health treatment plans showcased a paradigm shift, acknowledging that the mind and body are integral facets of well-being. The alliance between mental health professionals and fitness experts became a beacon of comprehensive care.

B. Emphasis on the Empowering Potential of Exercise for Mental Health

As we recap these key points, it is crucial to underscore the empowering potential that exercise carries for mental health. It is not merely a series of movements but a dynamic tool that individuals can wield to cultivate resilience, enhance mood, and foster a profound sense of well-being.

Exercise empowers individuals to take an active role in their mental health journey. It transcends the traditional boundaries of therapy and medication, offering a tangible and accessible avenue for individuals to reclaim agency over their well-being. The power lies not only in the physical exertion but in the intentional connection between the mind and body, creating a harmonious symphony of wellness.

C. Encouragement for Readers to Take the First Steps

As we conclude this journey, I extend a heartfelt encouragement to each reader. Take the first steps toward a healthier mind through physical activity. Embrace the understanding that your journey is unique, and the transformative power of exercise awaits your intentional engagement.

Start small, set realistic goals, and make exercise an enjoyable and sustainable part of your daily life. Whether it's a leisurely walk, a dance session, or a yoga practice, the choices are vast, and the possibilities are yours to explore. The journey toward a healthier mind begins with a single step— a step that holds the promise of resilience, vitality, and well-being.

In the tapestry of your life, let exercise be the vibrant thread that weaves a story of strength, renewal, and empowerment. As you embark on this transformative path, remember that you are not alone. The connection between exercise and mental health is a universal truth, and with each intentional stride, you join a community of individuals embracing the empowering potential of movement for the mind.

May your journey be filled with self-discovery, joy,
and the unwavering belief in your capacity to
cultivate a healthier and more resilient mind
through the simple yet profound act of exercise.